THE KETTLEBELL WORKOUT COMPANION

Dan John

Paperback: 978-1-963675-07-8

Published by OS Press

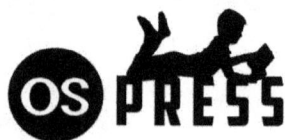

Contents

Contents

Foreword

I can honestly say that one of the secrets to any success I've had as a professional trainer and also as a person who strength trains is listening to and applying the wisdom of Dan John. Dan is a master at taking overly complex ideas about strength training and distilling them down into simple and effective practices. His books, lectures, and friendship have been instrumental in shaping the lens that I view strength training through.

What I really love about Dan is that he weighs and measures everything against results. If a training method yields effective results, he grades it and shares it for everyone to learn from. If a training method doesn't cut the mustard, he tosses it. He does this with the ideas and programs of others as well as with his own ideas and programs. In doing this, Dan is both the eager student and master teacher.

What you are holding in your hands is a book of tried and true kettlebell routines that will help you carve out and build the body you want to have. But more than that, its a book of training wisdom that has been accumulated, weighed, and tested through 60 years of training experience and over 45 years of coaching experience. What I'm saying is that you are holding GOLD in your hands. The last two pages alone are priceless. You can follow these routines and Dan's advice and build an amazingly strong body, for sure. BUT, you can also mine from these words and build an amazingly successful career as a coach, trainer, counselor, or teacher; or you can simply live a better life.

Tim Anderson

Co-founder of Original Strength and developer of the Pressing RESET method

Introduction

Not long ago, Zach Henderson asked me to do a simple workshop. "Hey Dan, can you go over some basic kettlebell workouts?" Sure, I said. Then, I started organizing my notes, workouts, books, and videos and realized that this would be a fun project. As I became more inspired, I kept adding more and more elements...and here we are with this "final" product.

I look forward to where this journey leads me in the kettlebell world. I was first exposed to kettlebells when the Soviet throwers (this was a while ago) were throwing these weird bowling balls with handles at the College of San Mateo. Kettlebells were originally measured in "poods," but it came across to Americans as "puds." You can still find throwing coaches using pud weights to increase the distance for the shot, discus, and hammer.

FIFTY years later, I am still exploring the art and science of kettlebell training. I hope you enjoy what you find here. Remember: it is in the exploration that you discover the hidden gems in training. One of my goals is to find ways to improve in all areas of my life. Sometimes, my searches take me in the wrong direction, but there are great lessons from mistakes. When I find things that work, I share them.

Some of these workout ideas and training sessions might not make sense while reading but will be perfectly clear in the doing. And... that's the best way to improve: DO! I can't sum this up better than what that famous coach, Yoda, taught us:

"Do. Or do not. There is no try."

Enjoy the doing. Enjoy the journey.

"Enough:" The Key to Kettlebell Training Sessions

At every Kettlebell certification, we discuss Kettlebells (KBs) for training sessions and long-term programming. Often, participants and their clients want "workouts," and there are thousands of options available in gyms, books, videos, and internet sites. Not all workouts are appropriate for every person and every "body."

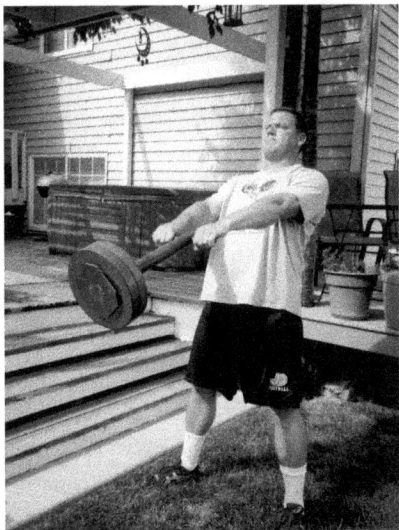

Dan trained swings with "kettlebell-like" objects before getting his first one. This was his "Hungarian Core Blaster" that allowed him to prep for his first KB certification.

Several times in my training life, I have had just a single KB as my entire gym. I was amazed to find this single bell is "enough." Enough to train my strength, challenge my conditioning, and help me be more mobile and flexible. As you approach planning and programming, use this marvelous tool, the kettlebell, to do more than just get you (or your clients or athletes) sweaty and hot.

No tool or training program is perfect. My highest standard is "Pretty Good," and KBs get that grade.

Important Note

Exercise has risks associated with it. Research shows it can lead to being stronger, healthier, and happier. However, it can also lead to injuries or even death. It happens.

You should also know that doing nothing also has risks associated with it. Research shows that being sedentary can lead to sickness, weakness, frailty, depression, and anxiety. It can also make you more injury-prone and hasten your destination towards death. It happens.

Consult your trusted family physician before beginning any exercise program or engaging in any sedentary lifestyle.

The Basic Basics: Bell Selection and the General Daily Outline

Let's first discuss a daily training session with an appropriate bell. For most men learning the KB world, the 20-kilogram bell is a good choice. For most women, the 10-kilogram bell is a good choice. Obviously, this little bit of advice is not a rule but a guideline. Many people will need to go heavier or lighter depending on age, experience, health, and goals. Let's get to work.

With the HKC (Hardstyle Kettlebell Challenge) Three (Swing, Goblet Squat, and Turkish Get-Up), we can challenge most people in a training program. Although less used today, the concept of the Minimum Effective Dose (the "MED" on some internet forums) still helps us design training days for ourselves, our clients, and our athletes. Here are the appropriate "doses" for the HKC Three:

Swings: 75-125 a day
Goblet Squats: 15-25 a day
Turkish Get-Ups: 1-10 each side a day.

If we add Push-Ups (15-25 a day), we might have a routine that will provide fitness, longevity, health, and performance. For many, this MED gets that Gold Standard of "Enough."

Yes, the devil is in the details. And…most people always want MORE when they should pursue ENOUGH.

Most of the time, for pure kettlebell workouts, do something like this for your training session:

- Naked (unweighted) Get-Ups for five minutes (Use partials as appropriate, too)
- Mobility Sequence (I use Original Strength's (Tim Anderson) Pressing RESET)
- Practice a few Hip Hinge Drills and a few Goblet Squat prying movements.
- Pick a KB workout. Time it, if appropriate.
- Turkish Get-Ups, one to five per side.
- Sparhawk or Cook Drill or Suitcase Carry or Waiter Walk as a Finisher.
- Rest, recover, repeat…in a day or so

Let's look at some of the KB workouts that I use.

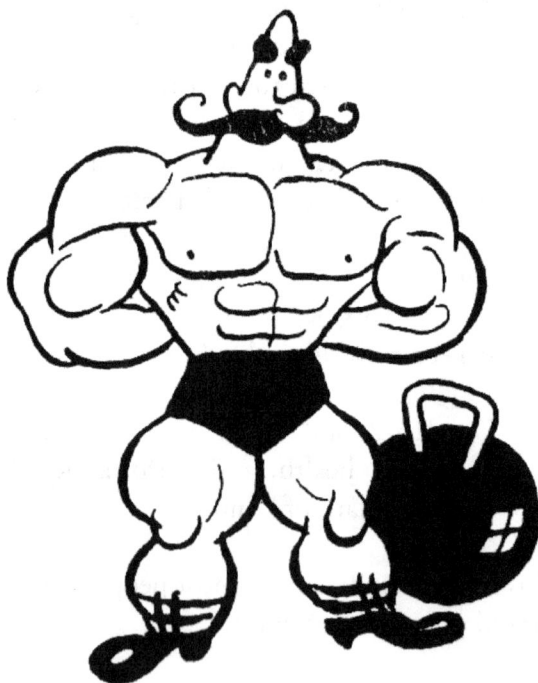

Bosco, Harry Paschall's creation, inspired a generation of lifters.
Used with permission from Bill Hinbern.

The First Twenty Days After Opening the Box with the New Kettlebell

I always worried that this First Twenty Days was "too much." However, I have received only positive reviews from our newly certified kettlebell instructors…and their clients.

The first twenty days after getting this new KB should be a chance to strive to master the movements and train the positions. Don't add speed and volume to poor movements: take your time to practice.

These twenty workouts can be done five days a week (a total of four weeks), three days a week (sneaking up on two months), or any way you choose. These will provide the grounding for a solid base. Strive for mastery.

Daily Warm Up

Many won't need much, but it is generally a good idea to go through some mobility drills, especially for these areas:

> Neck
> Shoulders
> Hips

Take one day each week to do a full "Toes to Top" mobility workout. In my gym, we use Original Strength's Pressing RESET as our core, whole-body approach to movement.

It is recommended that you do the Hip Flexor Stretch during each warm-up and cooldown period; it can be very well combined with an easy set of Goblet Squats. Many find a few easy sets of Swings, a few Goblet Squats, and a weightless set of one to five Get-Ups (both sides) to be enough warm-up.

Day One

3 Get-Ups Right
3 Get-Ups Left

Practice Hip Hinge
Goblet Squats: 2-3-5-2-3-5-2-3-5

Our First Training Session
      Five Two-Hand Swings
      One Goblet Squat
      Ten Reps of High Knee "March in Place" (Each time the right
      foot hits is "one rep")
      Recovery breathing (up to two minutes)
      For a total of Three Rounds

A few minutes of Pressing Practice.

Day Two

2 Get-Ups Right
2 Get-Ups Left
One-Hand Press (Start with "less strong arm" and alternate arms. "One
rep" is one arm right-hand press and one arm left-hand press)
1-2-3-1-2-3-1-2-3-1-2-3

Day Three

1 Get-Up Right
1 Get-Up Left

Today's Training Session
> Two-Hand Swings
> 30 Seconds of Swings
> 30 Seconds of Easy shaking of the arms and legs
> Twenty Minutes Total

Practice Goblet Squat

Day Four

10 Minutes of Get-Ups (Alternate Right and Left)

Today's Training Session
> Fifteen Two-Hand Swings
> One Goblet Squat
> Ten Reps of High Knee "March in Place" (Each time the right foot hits is "one rep")
> Recovery breathing (up to two minutes)
> For a total of Three Rounds

Day Five

5 Get-Ups Right
5 Get-Ups Left
One-Hand Press (Start with "less strong arm" and alternate arms. "One rep" is one arm right-hand press and one arm left-hand press)
1-2-3-1-2-3-1-2

Day Six

3 Minutes of Get-Ups (Alternate Right and Left)

Today's Training Session
   Two-Hand Swings
   30 Seconds of Swings
   30 Seconds of Easy shaking of the arms and legs
   Ten Minutes Total

Goblet Squat: Several sets of Five with a pause at the bottom

Day Seven

1 Get-Up Right
1 Get-Up Left
One-Hand Press (Start with "less strong arm" and alternate arms. "One rep" is one arm right-hand press and one arm left-hand press)
2-3-5-2-3-5-2-3-5

Day Eight

Ten Minutes of Get-Ups
Practice Hip Hinge
Practice Goblet Squat
Practice Press

Day Nine

1 Get-Up Right
1 Get-Up Left

Today's Training Session
    Fifteen Two-Hand Swings
    One Goblet Squat
    Ten Reps of High Knee "March in Place" (Each time the right foot hits is "one rep")
    Recovery breathing (up to two minutes)
    For a total of Five Rounds

One-Hand Press (Start with "less strong arm" and alternate arms. "One rep" is one arm right-hand press and one arm left-hand press)
1-2-3-1-2-3-1-2

Day Ten

5 Get-Ups Right
5 Get-Ups Left

Today's Training Session
    Two-Hand Swings
    30 Seconds of Swings
    30 Seconds of Easy shaking of the arms and legs
    Five Minutes Total

Goblet Squats
2-3-5-2-3-5

Day Eleven

5 Minutes of Get-Ups (Alternate Right and Left)
One-Hand Press (Start with "less strong arm" and alternate arms. "One rep" is one arm right-hand press and one arm left-hand press)
1-2-3-5-1-2-3-5-3

Today's Training Session
     Two-Hand Swings
     15 Seconds of Swings
     15 Seconds of "Fast Loose" Drills
     Ten Minutes Total

Day Twelve

Today's Training Session
     1 Get-Up Right
     1 Get-Up Left
     Two-Hand Swings
     30 Seconds of Swings
     30 Seconds of Easy shaking of the arms and legs
     Five Minutes Total

Goblet Squats
1-2-3-1-2-3-1-2

One-Hand Press (Start with "less strong arm" and alternate arms. "One rep" is one arm right-hand press and one arm left-hand press)
1-2-3-1-2-3-1-2

Day Thirteen

10 Minutes of Get-Ups (Alternate Right and Left)

Today's Training Session
    Fifteen Two-Hand Swings
    One Goblet Squat
    Ten Reps of High Knee "March in Place" (Each time the right foot hits is "one rep")
    Recovery breathing (up to two minutes)
    For a total of Ten Rounds

Day Fourteen

1 Get-Up Right
1 Get-Up Left
One-Hand Press (Start with "less strong arm" and alternate arms. "One rep" is one arm right-hand press and one arm left-hand press)
2-3-5-2-3-5-2-3-5

Day Fifteen

1 Get-Up Right
1 Get-Up Left

Today's Training Session
    Two-Hand Swings
    30 Seconds of Swings
    30 Seconds of Easy shaking of the arms and legs
    Five Minutes Total

Goblet Squats
1-2-3-1-2-3-1-2

One-Hand Press (Start with "less strong arm" and alternate arms. "One rep" is one arm right-hand press and one arm left-hand press)
1-2-3-1-2-3-1-2

Day Sixteen

Today's Training Session
> Fifteen Two-Hand Swings
> Five Goblet Squats
> *One Push Up*
> Ten Reps of High Knee "March in Place" (Each time the right foot hits is "one rep")
> Recovery breathing (up to two minutes)
> For a total of Ten Rounds

Day Seventeen

5 Minutes of Get-Ups (Alternate Right and Left)

One-Hand Press (Start with "less strong arm" and alternate arms. "One rep" is one arm right-hand press and one arm left-hand press)
2-3-5-2-3-5-2-3-5

Day Eighteen

3 Get-Ups Right
3 Get-Ups Left

Today's Training Session
> Two-Hand Swings
> 30 Second of Swings
> 30 Seconds of Easy shaking of the arms and legs
> Twenty Minutes Total

Day Nineteen

Goblet Squats
5-10-5-10-5

One-Hand Press (Start with "less strong arm" and alternate arms. "One rep" is one arm right-hand press and one arm left-hand press)
2-3-5-2-3-5-2-3-5

Day Twenty

1 Get-Up Right
1 Get-Up Left

Today's Training Session
Two-Hand Swings
30 Second of Swings
30 Seconds of Easy shaking of the arms and legs
Five Minutes Total

Goblet Squats
1-2-3-1-2-3-1-2

One-Hand Press (Start with "less strong arm" and alternate arms. "One rep" is one arm right-hand press and one arm left-hand press)
1-2-3-1-2-3-1-2

A Training Program in Ten Movements

I wrote this for my Godson, Seth. He only had a single bell in a dorm room. Later, Men's Health published this as its Workout of the Month. It's "pretty good" and a nice repeatable program for those who need a DO THIS program.

The movements, for the record:

1. **One-Arm Press**
2. **One-Arm row**
3. **Swing**
4. **Goblet Squat**
5. **Bird Dog**
6. **Push Up Position Plank (PUPP)**
7. **Hip Flexor Stretch**
8. **Hip Flexor Rainbows.**
9. **Six Point Zenith**
10. **Suitcase Carry**

Classical Conditioning in X Moves

My philosophy for strength training is based on three concepts:

1. Movements, not muscle
    The Fundamental Human Movements

    Push
    Pull
    Hinge
    Squat
    Loaded Carries
    The "Sixth Movement" includes everything else, from rolling to half-kneeling work to lunges. It also includes torque, twisting, rotational, and anti-rotational work.

2. "If it is important, do it every day; if it isn't, don't do it at all." This is a quote attributed to wrestling Olympic Gold Medalist Dan Gable.

    If we know the moves, how do we decide "when" to do them? I argue: every day. In my approach, we will explore the basic movements in nearly every workout. With most athletes, the movement needs repeating far more than most people think. At the elite levels of track and field and Olympic lifting, the total number of complete movements is simply staggering.

    "If it is important, do it every day; if it isn't, don't do it at all."

3. Repetitions...lots of repetitions.

Loading for the Program

A = Light(50%) / B = Medium(75%) / C = Heavy(100%)
For this program, the weight is **based on what you can do for ten repetitions**, not for a single lift. So, it will be a load that you can do "sometimes" for eight reps and sometimes for twelve, depending on things. Never miss a lift.

Program A – Simple Strength

Getting stronger is the foundation of all fitness goals. Stretching during rest periods keeps the intensity up (including heart rate). Strive to increase "C" over time.

Push One-Arm Press
- A x 10
  - o Hip Flexor Stretch Right Knee Down
- B x 5
  - o Hip Flexor Stretch Left Knee Down
- C x 10

Pull One-Arm Row
- A x 10
  - o Rainbow Right Knee Down
- B x 5
  - o Rainbow Left Knee Down
- C x 10

Hinge Swings
- A x 30
  - o Bird Dogs Right Knee Down
- B x 15
  - o Bird Dogs Left Knee Down
- C x 30

Squat Goblet Squat
- A x 10
  - o   Six Point Zenith right-hand Sweeps Up
- B x 5
  - o   Six Point Zenith left-hand Sweeps Up
- C x 10

Plank Push Up Plank (The goal is to build up to two minutes)

Carry Suitcase Carry. With the less dominant hand, walk as far as you can under load. Put the weight down. Turn around and come back with the dominant hand.

Program B – The Cardio Hit Workout

Mixing the dynamic swing with the grinding squat has been an interesting way to increase heart rate for the past few years. Adding the stretch between sets will keep the heart rate high but will also add some heart rate variability (a good thing). Don't hold the stretches for more than 30 Seconds; pop up for another set of swings.

- 15 Swings / One Goblet Squat
  - o   Hip Flexor Right Knee Down
- 15 Swings / One Goblet Squat
  - o   Hip Flexor Left Knee Down
- 15 Swings / One Goblet Squat
  - o   Rainbow Right Knee Down
- 15 Swings / One Goblet Squat
  - o   Rainbow Left Knee Down
- 15 Swings / One Goblet Squat
  - o   Bird Dog Right Knee Down
- 15 Swings / One Goblet Squat
  - o   Bird Dog Left Knee Down
- 15 Swings / One Goblet Squat
  - o   Six Point Zenith right-hand Sweeps Up

- 15 Swings / One Goblet Squat
  - Six Point Zenith left-hand Sweeps Up
- 15 Swings / One Goblet Squat
  - Push Up Plank
- 15 Swings / One Goblet Squat
  - Suitcase Walk R/L

Program C – Tonic Recharge Workout

This is the workout following a Tabata day. Yes, this is an easy day, but always focus on the long-term goal and the journey.

Push One Arm Press
- A x 10
  - Hip Flexor Right Knee Down
  - Hip Flexor Left Knee Down

Pull One Arm Row
- A x 10
  - Rainbow Right Knee Down
  - Rainbow Left Knee Down

Hinge Swings
- A x 30
  - Bird Dogs right Knee Down
  - Bird Dogs Left Knee Down

Squat Goblet Squat
- A x 10
  - Six Point Zenith right-hand Sweeps Up
  - Six Point Zenith left-hand Sweeps Up

Plank Push Up Plank
- 1:00

Program D - Bi - Monthly Tabata

Stay focused. It is only a ten-second rest, so be ready to go again in seven seconds. Go after it today. Please use a "Tabata Timer," available for free online. You go for twenty seconds, rest for ten, and repeat another seven times. (For a total of eight rounds and four minutes of working out)

- Tabata Workout One
  - Tabata Goblet Squats for 4 Minutes
- Tabata Workout Two
  - Tabata Swings for 4 Minutes

Program E - The Mobility Workout

Hold each position for thirty seconds.

- Under thirty years of age: go through the movements for two circuits (do every movement once, finish the list, repeat)
- From Thirty to Fifty: go through the movements for three circuits.
- Over fifty: At least three circuits; strive to do four or five.

Hip Flexor Right Knee Down
Hip Flexor Left Knee Down
Rainbow Right Knee Down
Rainbow Left Knee Down
Bird Dog Right Knee Down
Bird Dog Left Knee Down
Six Point Rainbow right-hand Sweeps Up
Six Point Rainbow left-hand Sweeps Up

For every lift or stretch:
- Ensure the feet are grounded: Stretch out the toes and grab the ground while driving the heels down.
- Whenever standing, attempt to level the belt of your pants parallel to the floor. Squeeze the Glutes to do this.
- Be sure to breathe! Mastery of breathing is one of the secrets to super strength.

One Arm Press
Use both hands to set the weight in place on the shoulder.
Squeeze your glutes first to begin the rep.
Strive to have the elbow in a vertical line under the wrist throughout the movement.
Finish with your beltline parallel to the floor.

One arm row
The non-working arm should be securely locked down on the off leg.
Hold the thumb of the working arm in the armpit for a short pause on every rep.
Do not jerk the weight. Move the weight under control and drive the elbow to the ceiling.

Swing
At the top of the movement, find the Plank position: glutes tight, thighs tight, and upper body tight. At the top, "throw" the weight back to the hinge.
Feel the "Hinge" in your hamstrings. Think of snapping a football back to a punter.

Squat
Begin the movement with the glutes locked and the belt line parallel. Drop the body between the legs and strive to push the knees OUT with the elbows. Pause. Squeeze the thighs to return to the standing position.

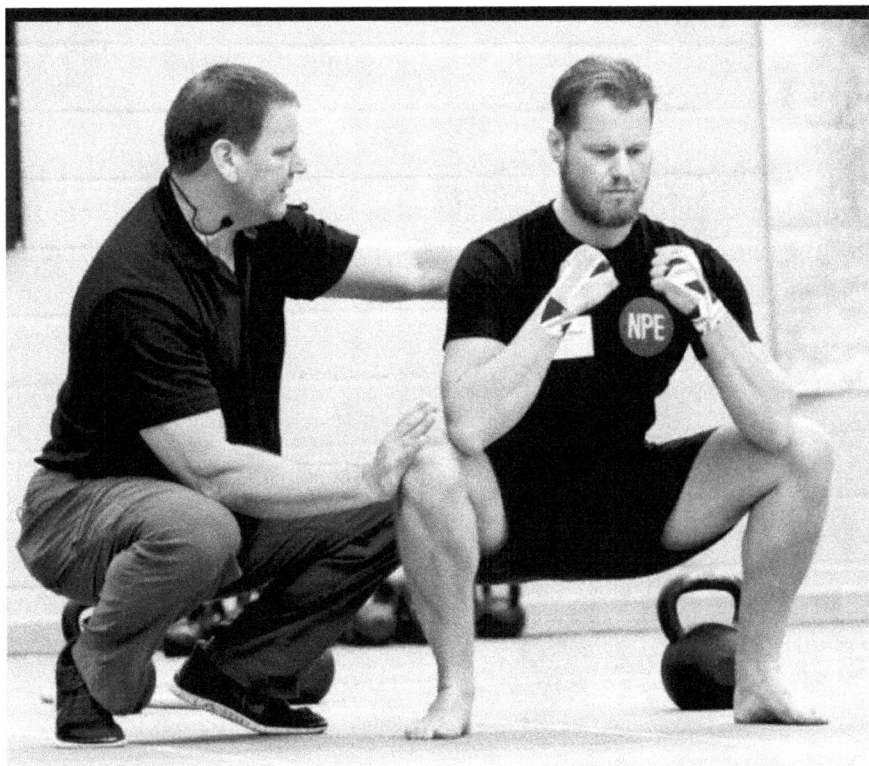

This picture, with James St. Pierre, might be the most popular Goblet Squat photograph ever taken. It has been used by countless websites.

Bird Dog

If the left knee is down, strive to drive the HEEL of the right foot straight back. Try to have both butt cheeks on the same plane parallel to the floor. Hold the Bird Dog for as long as you can. If you go over two minutes, pump the left elbow to the right knee for reps. Switch sides.

Push Up Position Plank (PUPP)

Squeeze the glutes. Try to squeeze "the heads of trolls" in your armpits. Hold this for up to two minutes. Focus on squeezing, not just surviving the time.

Planks, as a variation

Same as PUPP, but on the elbows. Try to pull the elbows to the knees throughout the time.

Hip Flexor Stretch

If the left knee is down, ensure the right big toe pushes hard into the ground. Squeeze the glutes and push the top of the head to Zenith. Feel the stretch in the left front hip. Switch sides.

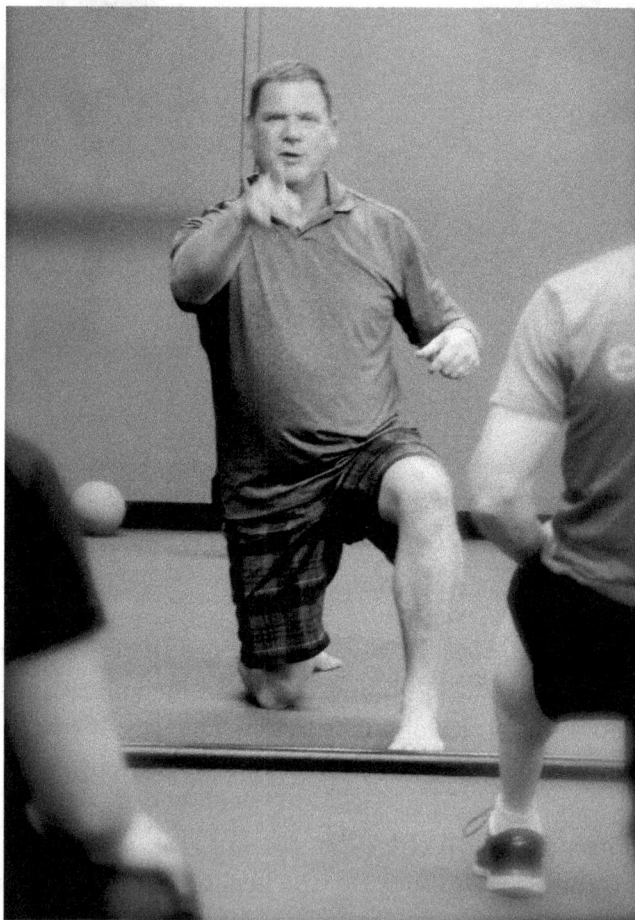

*Leading an impromptu session of fitness professionals
in the Half-Kneeling Hip Flexor Stretch.*

Hip Flexor Rainbows
The Hip Flexor Rainbows are the same, but with the left knee down, sweep the right arm in a long, slow arc from overhead to straight back, trying to open the chest and core.

Six Point Zenith
On your hands, knees, and feet (six-point), take your right arm and hug your left knee. Then, in a long, lazy arc, stretch the right arm up to Zenith or as close as you can. Use the same reach as the Hip Flexor Rainbow. Feel the stretch in your chest and core, and continue to hug and stretch.

Suitcase Carry
Pick up a weight in One-Hand. Stand tall, ensure your belt line is parallel, and walk. Repeat with the other side.

Sunday	Monday	Tuesday	Wednesday	Thursday	Friday	Saturday
	A Simple	E Mob	B Cardio		A Simple	D1 (GS)
	C (Tonic)	E Mob	A Simple		B Cardio	A Simple
	A Simple	E Mob	B Cardio		A Simple	D2 (Sw)
	C (Tonic)	E Mob	A Simple		B Cardio	A Simple

This is an excellent way of looping the workouts together. Having one day a week, Tuesday in this example, to do just mobility work is a nice way to keep any program fresh. Please note that we do Simple Strength twice a week and six Cardio (four "B Cardios" and the Tabata Days) workouts a month. Most people need to get their strength and hypertrophy (lean body mass) improved, although I found the Tabatas to do a lot for LBM. I like having two days off a week to enjoy life.

Don't ignore the Tonic workouts. Many people err by missing a chance to move and refresh. It's part of an intelligent, long-term approach to training, but many ignore the simple Tonic workouts that are the "hair of the dog that bit you."

The Single KB Workout Family

The following are the classic workouts that I have used for almost two decades. They are popular worldwide.

The Humane Burpee (Thanks to Dan Martin for the name!)

Be sure to follow the advice about reps on the Goblet Squat (GS) and Push-Up: We want the reps to descend as we move through the Humane Burpee, hence the name.

So, here you go:

15 Swings
5 Goblet Squats
5 Push-Ups

15 Swings
4 Goblet Squats
4 Push-Ups

15 Swings
3 Goblet Squats
3 Push-Ups

15 Swings
2 Goblet Squats
2 Push-Ups

15 Swings
1 Goblet Squat
1 Push-Up

That's 75 swings, 15 Goblet Squats, and 15 Push-Ups. The real exercise is popping up and down for the Push-Ups. Most of us don't take any rest at all during the workout but feel free to stop when you need to rest.

The real exercise is popping up and down for the Push-Ups.

To make it more challenging, just slide the Goblet Squats and Push Ups up to ten. 10-9-8-7-6-5-4-3-2-1 gives you 55 total reps, which is plenty of work for a single day....in many cases, it is too much.

Here are three other variations that have value.

I don't remember why I called these "**Slurpees,**" but I did. This one is a good conditioner.

10 or 15 Swings
5 Goblet Squats
10 Mountain Climbers (every time the left foot hits is a rep).

Let the GSs descend (5-4-3-2-1). That gives you 50-75 Swings, 15 GS, and a lot of heart-pounding.

Hornees

Hornees are the first of our Loaded Carries training sessions. A Horn Walk is simply walking around with the bell on the chest (the hands hold the horns...get it?). It keeps the tension high. So:

10 or 15 Swings
5 Goblet Squats
Horn Walk for an appropriate distance.

Again, let the GSs descend (5-4-3-2-1). That gives you 50-75 Swings, 15 GS, and an interesting feeling in the whole area of muscles that squeeze things together.

Bearpees (great in groups)

10 or 15 Swings
5 Goblet Squats
Bear Crawl

Again, descend with the GS (5-4-3-2-1). In groups, you can have the two people be 60 feet apart, and share the same bell. You will see a lot of racing here, and the participants will quickly learn that they underestimate the crawling.

The Coyote

This workout is a staple of the Coyote Point Kettlebell Club. It takes only one Kettlebell per person and can be adjusted with reps, sets, and load to fit anyone. Don't let the simplicity fool you:

15 Swings
5 Goblet Squats
3 Push Ups (or variations)

This little workout covers all the basic human movements and has the odd ability to allow "one more round." Simply try this for five rounds the first time, and you will find it appropriate and repeatable. If you can handle the volume, 20 rounds become 300 swings, 100 squats, and 60 Push-Ups, and that is a respectable workout.

To make it more challenging, increase the Push-Ups first, then add a bigger bell. This is a great workout anywhere, any time, for any reason.

The 10,000 Swing Challenge

Years ago, my friends at T-Nation asked me for a doable but hard challenge with kettlebells. I thought 20 workouts of 500 swings would fit the idea of a challenge. It became an internet phenomenon. So, 20 workouts (in a row, five times a week, four times a week, whatever you like) of 500 swings = 10,000 swings. I like to do this five times a week…making it a four-week challenge.

The simplest version is this:

Swing 10 reps
One Goblet Squat
Swing 15 reps
Two Goblet Squats
Swing 25 reps
Three Goblet Squats
Swing 50 reps

Rest. That is 100 repetitions, so just swim through these four more times (five total giant sets). (Next time, do push-ups, pull-ups, ab wheels, or whatever.)

Later, Mike Warren Brown and I designed these kinds of workouts where you just pick strength or mobility moves to get 250 swings "easily." Don't worry about the names of anything (most are demonstrated on my YouTube channel or danjohnuniversity.com). In fact, I encourage you to design options based on your equipment and ideas/needs.

Group A
1. 35 Swings
2. Push-Ups
3. 15 Swings
4. Windmill Stick Right
5. 35 Swings
6. TRX T Pull
7. 15 Swings
8. Windmill Stick Left
9. 35 Swings
10. Trap Bar DL
11. 15 Swings
12. Stoney Stretch Right Knee Down (RKD)
13. 35 Swings
14. Goblet Squat
15. 15 Swings
16. Stoney Stretch Left Knee Down (LKD)
17. 35 Swings
18. Rolling 45s
19. 15 Swings
20. "Pump" Downward Dog/Cobra

Group B
1. 35 Swings
2. One-Arm Press Right Arm
3. 15 Swings
4. TRX Long Stretch Right
5. 35 Swings
6. One-Arm Press Left Arm
7. 15 Swings
8. TRX Long Stretch Left
9. 35 Swings
10. TRX Y Pull
11. 15 Swings
12. Hip Flexor Stretch (RKD)

13. 35 Swings
14. Goblet Squat
15. 15 Swings
16. Hip Flexor Stretch (LKD)
17. 35 Swings
18. Rolling 45 Ts
19. 15 Swings
20. March in Place

LKD=Left Knee Down. RKD=Right Knee Down

An interesting version with the Turkish Get-Up will really get your heart pumping (oddly enough, groundwork seems to increase HR):

Swing 10 reps
One TGU, weight in left-hand
Swing 15 reps
One TGU, weight in right-hand
Swing 25 reps
Two TGUs, one left and one right
Swing 50 reps

A small note: I always go "Left First" when it comes to any One-hand, one-leg, or one-foot movement. That way, one never needs to remember what to do next. Ignore this at your own peril with large groups.

Single KB Loaded Carry Workouts

I name Loaded Carry workouts after the birds of the Raptor family. It started as a joke about how we are picking up things and moving them, but we soon found that this was a nice way of organizing them. This workout is called the Sparrow Hawk or **Sparhawk**.

You will be doing Goblet Squats and Suitcase Carries. Suitcase Carries are like Farmer Walks, but you only load one side…like you are carrying a single suitcase.

It's simple:
8 Goblet Squats, then march away with the bell in the left hand about 60 feet (gym length is best)
7 Goblet Squats, then return to the original position with the bell in the right hand
6 Goblet Squats, left-hand suitcase walk
5 Goblet Squats, right-hand walk
4 Goblet Squats, left-hand walk
3 Goblet Squats, right-hand walk
2 Goblet Squats, left-hand walk
1 Goblet Squat, finished

That is 36 squats, but you are under load for about three minutes. So, your anti-rotation muscles will be working overtime with the asymmetrical walking and will still have to join in to support the squats. You get the benefits of squatting, including the mobility and flexibility work, plus the additional boon of three minutes of time under tension.

Next, consider the "**Cook Drill**" from Gray Cook, P.T., founder of the Functional Movement System.

Here's how it works: Stand and hold a kettlebell in the rack.

Now press the bell straight overhead and walk. This is the Waiter Walk. Your arm should be completely straight, and your shoulder "packed" (pull it down, away from your ear).

If you feel your arm start to wobble or your core starts to shift, you've lost integrity. When that happens, bring the weight back to the rack position. Hold this position and continue to walk until you feel yourself losing integrity again. Release the weight to your side so you're holding it like a suitcase. Once you can't hold the weight in that position, switch hands and start from the beginning.

Gray recommends this for up to 15 minutes, but we get plenty with just going about 400 meters. What am I saying? We did that ONCE. We usually don't go very long, but occasionally, this is a great drill all by itself.

The Road Warrior

This is a workout I designed for federal agency members who travel frequently and never know what equipment they will have available. It is simple on paper but keeps your conditioning "in the ballpark" until you come stateside again.

Symmetrical Workouts

Day One

> With KB (or dumbbell) in one hand ONLY (Let's say left hand)
>
> Waiter Walk (Short walk around with weight overhead like a waiter)
> Suitcase Carry (Short walk around with weight like a suitcase)

Suitcase Deadlifts (Hinge Movement, One-sided deadlifts)
One-Hand Presses Overhead
One-Hand Bench Presses (Keep other hand "free")
Side Bends

Repeat for as many sets as appropriate.

Day Two

Do Day One's workout with the other hand!

Reps and sets depend on the weight available (and energy available). Get it going and feel good.

Day Three

Combine Push Ups and Swings (or any variation)
Swings 20
Push Ups 5
Swings 20
Push Ups 4
Swings 20
Push Ups 3
Swings 20
Push Ups 2
Swings 20
Push Ups 1
Swings 20
Repeat or adjust as appropriate.

The Single KB Armor Building Complex

I stand by my version of the single bell ABC. It's reasonable. Here you go:

- Left hand: One clean and press
- *Switch hands*
- right hand: One clean and press
- Immediately followed by two single-side KB front squats
- *Bell down to the ground. Shake out your arms and legs a moment and…go!*
- right hand: One clean and press
- *Switch hands*
- left hand: One clean and press
- Immediately followed by two single-side KB front squats

And that is "One."

When added up, it is four cleans, four presses, and four front squats. It contains the elements of the classic kettlebell workouts from the early days of the 2000s when most people just had one KB and strived to find ways to utilize the tool better. The math is easy for volume:

10 Rounds = 40 Cleans, 40 Presses, 40 Front Squats

20 Rounds = 80 Cleans, 80 Presses, 80 Front Squats

30 Rounds = 120 Cleans, 120 Presses, 120 Front Squats (and…ouch, the stairs are going to hurt)

Two Kettlebell Workouts

The **Armor Building Complex**, the ABC, was initially called the "Grad Workout." I came up with this workout after it became apparent that KB cert weekends needed to finish with a training session that didn't hurt people. There **were some** *issues,* and I spent some time working on the answer. Here are the issues:

1. We have an exhausted cadre.
2. Putting bells up overhead with exhausted people breaks all the safety rules.
3. Some people have little skin on their hands by the last day.
4. Any idiot can get people tired. Getting people to test themselves under stress and exhaustion takes some thinking to keep things safe.

With these problems/opportunities, I reached into my grab bag of training and came up with this simple workout:

Double Kettlebell Clean for two reps
Double Kettlebell Press for one rep
Double Kettlebell Front Squat for three reps.
Put the bell down like a professional. Step away.

Now, your partner takes the bells while you do easy shaking of the arms and legs and support the community as you can.

Repeat. A lot.

In my book, the Armor Building Formula, trainees alternate one day of ABCs with one day of high repetition pressing. The formula for pressing is:

2 reps…appropriate rest
3 reps…appropriate rest

5 reps…a bit more rest
10 reps, and the round finishes. That's 20 reps.

Five rounds builds up to 100 reps. Whether you use double KB presses or singles is up to you and your equipment. Single bells do take longer, but the load is half. So, as I sadly say too often, it depends. I like pressing in all its forms, so I don't mind rotating exercises from week to week and experimenting with chasing fatigue.

One of the issues with the ABF that keeps coming up is loading the high-rep press days. For some people, our "born pressers," this isn't an issue. For others, including several people I work with daily, we have had to make some simple adjustments.

One difficulty in selecting weights for presses or giving advice about what loads to use in any exercise is that we have lots of wonderful people lifting weights, which vary in gender, age, experience, genetics, interests, passion, and goals. One size fits all is what a lot of people want to sell you, but a few months in a typical gym will show that there are no formulas to make this work. I wrote the following years ago, and I want to share this with you before we move on to basic math.

It is hard for most of us to understand the level of commitment it takes to achieve the highest levels of a sport.

It is hard for most of us to understand the level of commitment it takes to achieve the highest levels of a sport. In the weight room, we might need a decade to approach our best lifts. As I covered in my book *Never Let Go*, we have four kinds of maximal performance:

1. Sorta Max: This is something I can do without any thought or effort. It's what most people think they can do.
2. Max: If someone special shows up while I'm training or I travel to another place and am spurred on by others or some charismatic coach, this would be my "best."

3. Max Max: This would be what I could do if I plotted and planned a performance for at least six months or a year.
4. Max Max Max: This is that effort that I guarantee has a story behind it. It's for a win, a championship, or a lifesaving effort. Most people who hit this level probably doubt that they could repeat it.

To help followers of the ABF deal with the Sorta Max to probably Max range, I plugged in Boyd Epley's old formula from the 1980s of using reps with a weight to figure out, in a general sense, one's one rep max. No formula is perfect, and many of us discover this in competitions: You might be a lot stronger than you think when you want to win a contest!

This is the formula:
1RM = weight x (1 + (reps / 30))

Thank you, Brad Pilon, for reminding me about this, as it really is something to consider.

Reps	8 K Bell	10 K Bell	12 K Bell	16 K Bell	20 K Bell	24 K Bell	32 K Bell	Reps
1	8	10	12	16	20	24	32	1
2	8	10	12	16	20	24	32	2
3	8	10	12	16	20	24	32	3
4	8	10	12	16	20	24	36*	4
5	8	12	14	18*	20	28*	36	5
6	10	12	14	18	24	28	36	6
7	10	12	14	18/20*	24	28	36/40*	7
8	10	12	14	20*	24	28	40	8
9	10	12	16	20	24	28	40	9
10	10	12	16	20	24	32	40	10
11	10	12/14*	16	22*	28*	32	44*	11
12	10	14*	16	22	28	32	44	12
13	10	14	16	22	28	32	44	13
14	12	14	18*	22	28	32	44	14
15	12	14	18	24	28	36*	48*	15

We use this chart in my gym to help pick loads for people who struggle with the fives and tens sets. It's not perfect, but if you can press the 32 for reps 2-3-5 but flail going higher, drop to the 24 for your ten reps and enjoy. I've received some fun feedback from people playing around with "max attempts" with those high-rep presses. Pressing big weights for 15 might not be for everyone, but it sure is a fun challenge.

Remember that: "It's a fun challenge." Training should be fun, too.

One other thing: When KBs first returned to the public eye just after the year 2000 or so, only three sizes were available. I LIKED that, as it forced people to train and learn with an appropriate load before trying to go up heavier. Let me share the numbers if you have just the classic three (16, 24, and 32-kilogram kettlebells).

Reps	16 K Bell	24 K Bell	32 K Bell
1	16	24	32
2	16	24	32
3	16	24	32
4	16	24	32
5	16	24	32
6	16	24	32
7	16	24	32
8	16	24	32
9	16	24	32
10	16	32	32
11	16	32	32
12	16	32	32
13	16	32	32
14	16	32	32
15	24	32	32

As you can see, you need to handle some serious reps before testing the bigger bell IF you only have the three originals. For the record, this is one of the reasons I liked the simplicity of these three.

As always, seek some challenges in your training.

The EAGLE

A few years ago, I discovered the combination I call The Eagle. The school mascot where I was teaching at the time was the Soaring Eagle, so the name was natural. It combined the simplest of the loaded carries—the patterning movement of the farmer walk—with the basic grinding squat, the double-kettlebell front squat.

I will say 'simply' here, but the workload is incredible. Simply, the athletes do eight double-kettlebell front squats, then drop the weight to their sides and farmer walk for 20 meters, then they do another eight squats and repeat until they complete eight circuits.

The load for a high school male is 24 kg per hand. Females can do the 12s.

The goal was often not met.

There are some hidden benefits to this combo. The athlete needs two kettlebells and never puts them down. The metabolic hit is accelerated by the grip work, the wrestling with the kettlebells, and the sheer volume of carrying the load. It was this Eagle that made me think about the ideal combos.

There is nothing magical in the choice of exercises; it is simply the patterning movement of loaded carries mixed with the grinding movement of squats. For whatever reason, those two kettlebells are also a sign from heaven that this will be a hard workout.

Finally, on Loaded Carries, use your imagination. I've been inventing fun variations for decades now, and all of them have value. This photo on the next page, taken by Mark Twight, shows me doing the Farmer Walk backward, dragging a sled. It's wonderful for the knees and for your neighbors to watch.

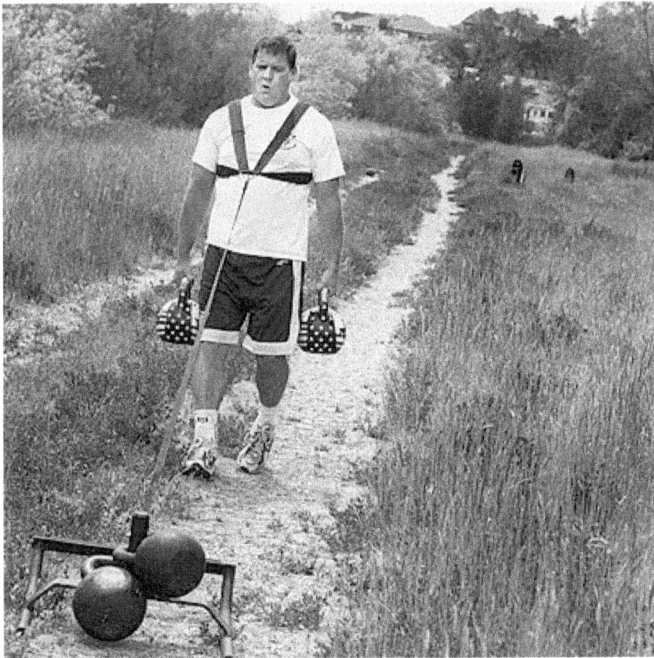

Multiple Kettlebell Workouts

Conga Lines

Dun-dun-dun-dun-dun-DA!

That's about as well as I can do with music. Conga lines! Stretch out every KB you have in a line, circle, or down the street like we do. Pick a lift. Do a single. Step to the next bell. Do a single. Continue. If you have 35 bells, that's a lot of reps.

A few things: I recommend only using odd numbers of bells so you can start with the left hand. When you come around to the start, start with the right hand so you keep the left to right in balance.

Next, do NOT go in any order with the KB weights. Now, we tend to go medium-heavy-light with three bells, but that is the only time we think about it. Make it as random as possible. There is nothing like clean and pressing the 48 and then taking the 4-kilogram bell. I think it teaches control. Here are some fun ideas:

- Goblet squats
- Single side squats
- Clean and press (probably the best for most situations)
- Snatches (these are good if you have lots of snatch-sized bells)

Let your imagination flow, but most people think the clean and press works best. One can also MAKE an exercise work by simply having three or five reasonable bells and go through multiple times, like with the snatch.

Don't overthink it. Put the bells out and go. Learn from your mistakes or successes and do it again soon.

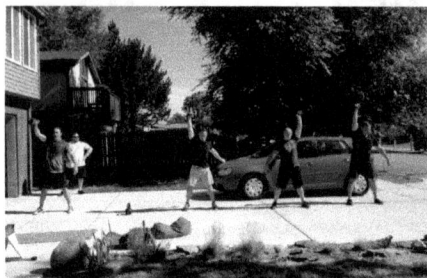

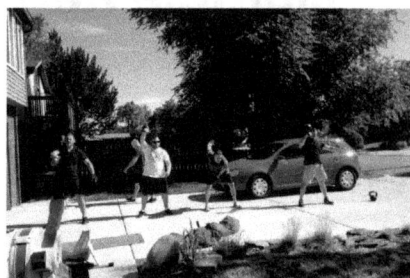

This is my Intentional Community from a few years ago. We are doing Clean and Press with five KBs, and...try this. It's a lot of work in a reasonable, repeatable, and doable fashion.

The Turkish Get-Up!

First, the "Why" of TGUs

Otto Arco, at a body weight of 138 pounds, could do a One-Hand Get-Up with 175 pounds. The Get-Up was his "secret" to all-around body strength, power, and composition. Arco wrote this in his book, "How to Learn Muscle Control"

> *The main purpose of muscle-control is self-mastery. Muscle control involves far more than the mere ability to make the muscles contract. It teaches you to relax, which is sometimes even more important than contraction. It gives you selective control and, therefore, the ability to single out those muscles necessary to the work to be done and only those muscles, leaving the antagonistic, or non-helpful, muscles relaxed.*

> *That makes a saving of energy in two ways; since it enables you to put all your energy into stimulating the needed muscles, and relieves those muscles of the interference of needlessly flexed antagonistic muscles. Muscle control, which leads to body-control, is great factor for success in all competitive sports.*

Arco, over a century ago, singles out the core and keys to the use of kettlebells: "Selective Control." This is the ability to turn to stone when necessary and when to relax…when necessary! It is the secret behind Bruce Lee's One Inch Punch and the ability to hit a golf ball far. (And, more importantly, throw the discus far.)

The Get Back UP
(Introducing the TGU without Load)

Doctor Claudio Gil Araújo, who performed a study at Clinimex-Exercise Medicine Clinic in Rio de Janeiro, said being able to stand up from a seated position on the ground was "remarkably predictive" of physical strength, flexibility and coordination at a range of ages. Araújo said: "If a middle-aged or older man or woman can sit and rise from the floor using just One-Hand—or even better without the help of a hand—they are not only in the higher quartile of musculo-skeletal fitness but their survival prognosis is probably better than that of those unable to do so."

Each of the two basic movements is assessed (to the ground and back to standing) and scored out of five, making a composite score of ten, with one point subtracted per support, such as a hand or knee, used. Here is the interesting part: Those who scored three points or fewer had a five to six times higher risk of death than those scoring more than eight points. A score below eight was linked with two to fivefold higher death rates over the 6.3-year study period.

Doctor Araújo said, "Our study also shows that maintaining high levels of body flexibility, muscle strength, power-to-body weight ratio and coordination are not only good for performing daily activities but have a favorable influence on life expectancy."

One thing I have realized is that many Americans literally spend no time on the ground. So, I came up with a little teaching drill that masquerades as a cardiovascular workout for some and a mobility workout for others. It's called "Get Back Ups," or GBUps.

There's an important key to using this drill: Do not overcoach. In fact, intentionally undercoach the whole movement.

Announce the position on the ground (on the front, on the right side, on the left side, pushup position plank, and on the back). Wait for the client, or clients, to get in position. When all have stopped moving, announce, "Get back up." When all are standing still, move to the next position.

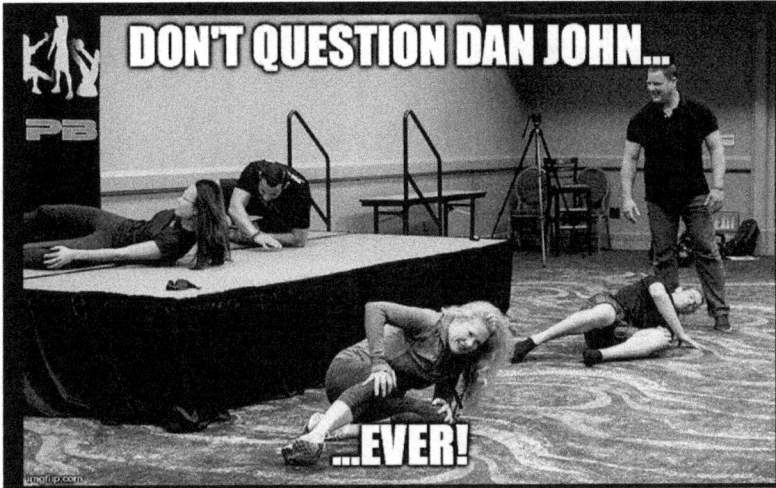

This picture is from a Perform Better event and someone turned it into a meme. My sister, Corinne, sent it to me and wondered why people pay money to see me.

Series One
The hands are free.
- On your front (or on your belly)
- Get back up
- On your right side
- Get back up
- On your left side
- Get back up
- Pushup position plank
- Get back up
- On your back
- Get back up

Series Two

The right hand is stuck to the right knee (tell them a puppy dies if their hands come loose from their knees).

- On your front (or on your belly)
- Get back up
- On your right side
- Get back up
- On your left side
- Get back up
- Pushup position plank
- Get back up
- One your back
- Get back up

Series Three

The left hand is stuck to the left knee

- On your front (or on your belly)
- Get back up
- On your right side
- Get back up
- On your left side
- Get back up
- Pushup position plank
- Get back up
- On your back
- Get back up

Series Four

*The right hand is stuck to the **left knee.***

- On your front (or on your belly)
- Get back up
- On your right side
- Get back up
- On your left side
- Get back up
- Pushup position plank

- Get back up
- On your back
- Get back up

Series Five
*The left hand is stuck to the **right knee.***
- On your front (or on your belly)
- Get back up
- On your right side
- Get back up
- On your left side
- Get back up
- Pushup position plank
- Get back up
- On your back
- Get back up

Note: I also use "Both hands in the back pocket," "Hands behind the head," and "Hands on shoulders" for variety. The PUPP still stays, and it's enlightening to see how the person attempts to do these.

Doing all five series is a total of twenty-five reps of going up and down, and the group will be hot and sweating. It's a fine warm-up, but it also seems to improve movement. As the movements are restricted (hands on knees), the client needs to develop new strategies to get back up and down.

T-Spine Mobility for the Hinging and Twisting Lifts

This is my progression I teach at all KB certs and some workshops. It's a blend of Original Strength's (Tim Anderson) Pressing RESET and the classic movements of the KB world.) It's beyond this work's scope to explain the Windmill and Bent Press, but they teach a lot about the human body…under load.

Prone
       Neck Nods
       Find Your Shoes
       Pumps
       Egg Rolls (Same as Windmills/BP)
Six Point
       Rocks
       Nods
       Find Your Shoes
       Big Hip Circles
       Figure 8s
       Cat-Cow
Eight Point
       Circles
Tall Kneeling
       Egyptians (SeeSaw like BP)
Standing with Sticks
       Dislocates
       Figure 8s

"Unwind and Unhinge"
    Wide Stance Windmill
    Windmill Sticks
    Narrow Stance Windmills
Kneeling Windmill
    Pump (1/2 Kneeling to KW)
    KW: Elbow to Ground
    KW "Hand Off" Windmill
Standing
    Wide Stance Windmill
    RKC Windmill (*Just twist feet*)
        All three: overhead, ground, double
Kettlebells
    TGU Press

Load and Strength Standards for Life...and Kettlebells

Survive before Thrive

Stand on One Foot for Ten Seconds
Hang from a Bar for 30 seconds
SLJ your Body Height (for distance, not height!)
Squat down, hold for 30 seconds, and Stand Up.
Farmers Walk Bodyweight for X Distance ("X" means you should be able to pick up your bodyweight, walk literally "whatever," a few steps is fine, and put it back down)
Keep your "GetBackUp" Test at 8

Men's Standards

Paul Lyngso shared these with me years ago, and they stand the test of time.

Squat Movement
1. Proper Form in the Goblet Squat
2. Goblet Squat: 24K x 10
3. Double KB Front Squat: 32K x 10
4. Bodyweight Back Squat
5. Bodyweight Front Squat
6. Bodyweight Back Squat x 15
7. Bodyweight Overhead Squat x 15

Hip Hinge Movement
1. Hip Hinge with Proper Form (From stand, floor and loaded)
2. Kettlebell Swing: 24K x 20 (Proper Form)
3. Double KB Clean: 32K x 10
4. Barbell Clean: Bodyweight
5. Barbell Deadlift: Double Bodyweight
6. Barbell Snatch: Bodyweight
7. Barbell Deadlift 2.5 x Bodyweight

Press Movement
1. Push Ups x 10
2. One Arm KB Press: 24K x 5 per Side
3. Double Press: 32K x 5
4. Bench Press: Bodyweight
5. One Arm Overhead Press: ½ Bodyweight
6. Bench Press: Bodyweight x 15
7. Two Arm KB Press: Bodyweight

Pull Movement
1. Batwings, thumbs in armpits, 16K x 10 seconds
2. Bodyweight Row on Rings/TRX x 20
3. Bodyweight Row, feet elevated, x 10
4. Chin Ups x 5
5. Pull Ups x 8-10
6. Pull Ups x 15
7. Weighted Pull Up with 48K

Women's Standards

Squat Movement
1. Proper Form in the Goblet Squat
2. Goblet Squat: 12K x 10
3. Double KB Front Squat: 16K x 5
4. Back Squat: 135 x 5
5. Bodyweight Back Squat
6. Bodyweight Front Squat
7. Bodyweight Overhead Squat

Hip Hinge Movement
1. Hip Hinge with Proper Form (From stand, floor and loaded)
2. Kettlebell Swing: 16K x 20 (Proper Form)
3. Double KB Clean: 16K x 10
4. Barbell Deadlift: 1.5 x Bodyweight (or 135 x 5)
5. Double KB Swings: 24K x 10
6. Bodyweight Clean
7. Barbell Deadlift 2 x Bodyweight (or, simply, 275lbs.)

Press Movement
1. Push Ups x 1 (Excellent Pushup)
2. One-Arm KB Press: 10K x 5 per Side
3. Double KB Press: 12K x 5
4. Double KB Press: 16K x 5
5. One-Arm Overhead Press: ⅓ Bodyweight
6. Bench Press: Bodyweight
7. Two-Arm KB Press: 2/3 Bodyweight

Pull Movement
1. Batwings, thumbs in armpits, 8K x 10 seconds
2. Bodyweight Row on Rings/TRX x 20
3. Bodyweight Row, feet elevated, x 10
4. Chin Ups x 1
5. Chin Ups x 3
6. Pull Ups x 3
7. Weighted Pull-Up with 24K

The Original RKC II Standards
(Only discussed, never used)

<u>Men</u>
Press the Beast
Snatch 24 kg bell 200 times in ten minutes

<u>Women</u>
Press the 24 kg bell
Snatch the 16 kg bell 200 times in ten minutes
(Both tests should be done in under 30 minutes)

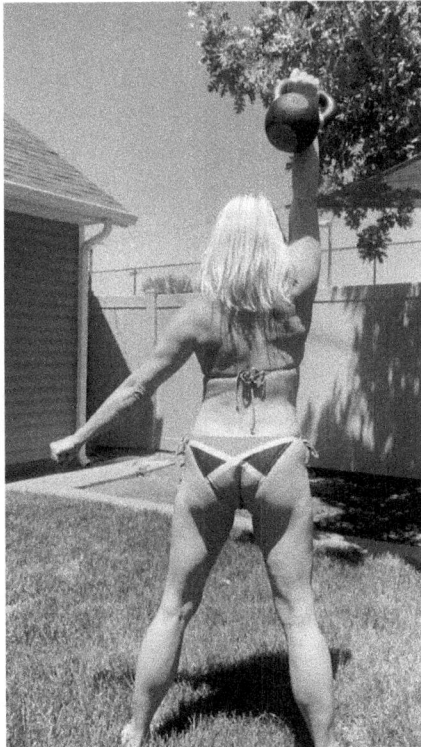

One of my best clients - a 55-year-old woman who takes heavy KBs seriously.

Some Numbers to Think About

- Waistline Numbers
  - Men
    - Under 37 inches: Healthy
    - Between 37 and 40 inches: Some Health Risks
    - Over 40 inches: Clear Health Risks
  - Women
    - Under 31 inches: Healthy
    - Between 31 and 35 inches: Some Health Risks
    - Over 35 inches: Clear Health Risks
- Waist Height (Healthy Numbers)
  Lay on your back and have someone with a ruler measure how high your waist is at its peak.
  - Men: Under 8.7 inches
  - Women: Under 7.9 inches

The Basics of Long-Term Planning (Programming)

The key to planning anything is to "start here" and have some idea of where you want to finish. I believe Yogi Berra said: "If you don't know where you are going, any road will take you there." In my experience, and I was first informed of this by the work of Earl Nightingale, only about five percent of the population has any interest in physical activity. If you are reading this, I am confident you are a "five percenter."

I started lifting in 1965, and I don't see a finish line, but I now have shorter goals based on my values. I cover this concept of values training in my *Inner Circle Group*. I'm not cross-selling here, but it takes about twelve weeks to cover the concept of values-based goals. I still compete as an Olympic lifter, so I often have short-term goals that support my key values of fitness and order.

We have a key principle in our gym: 5 x 52. It's simple: five workouts a week, every week of the year. How you go about that is a lot like deciding what's for dinner: you have a buffet of options. I always tell people when it comes to planning training that "pretty good" is my highest standard. Don't strive for perfect: get the training sessions in, week in and week out, and collect the benefits.

Here are a few ideas for you:

1. Follow every training session with a walk. If you need to use a treadmill, exercise bike, or other device, that's fine, too. I strive for 30–45-minute walks after every workout.
2. For most people, most of the time, lifting three days a week is going to be optimal. If you are the proud owner of KBs in your

home, you can add more days of variety and exploration, but keep the lifting (most people, most of the time) to three days a week.

3. I strongly encourage a single session a week to explore mobility and flexibility. We do ours on Thursdays, aka "Tonic Thursdays."

4. I also like one longer walking session a week. We load up with vests or weighted backpacks and we also Heavy Hand. An hour or so doing this seems to bring the sweat out, no matter the temperature. A long hike on the weekend might have benefits far beyond the exercise.

5. Review the "Ten Commandments" (see below) and realize it's okay to have variations, changes, missteps, and pure astonishment as you train for weeks, months, years, and decades.

If you decide to train with KBs three times a week, I suggest a simple A-B-A, then B-A-B approach. For example:

"A" workouts can be the strength movements ("grinds"). For most KB enthusiasts, it would be the press, squat, and get-up family. For my Armor Building Formula (ABF), I emphasize the half-kneeling presses (up to 100 total reps). As I age, the benefits of the overhead presses and the intense glute work of KBs have become my fountain of youth.

"B" workouts, for example, can be challenges or complexes. With the ABF, we do lots of rounds of the double kettlebell Armor Building Complex. I suggest, after a short break-in period of two or three weeks, to alternate weeks with one session of complexes one week followed by two sessions the next.

Adding a tonic day and maybe an extra day or two a week of adding walking and mobility work is a repeatable, doable, and reasonable approach to training for "most of us, most of the time."

A Two-Week Example

The key to this is that it is an EXAMPLE. This is a good example of a two-week template. It's best to dive in, experiment, practice, and take good notes on your training. After about two weeks, you will have a better sense of what you need to do more (or less) of in your training.

Week One

Monday
- Naked (unweighted) Turkish Get-Ups for five minutes
- Mobility Sequence
- Practice a few Hip Hinge Drills and a few Goblet Squat prying movements.
- Humane Burpee or Armor Building Challenge
- Turkish Get-Ups, one to five per side.
- Sparhawk
- Walk

Tuesday
- GetBackUps
- Mobility Sequence
- Walk, Ruck, or HeavyHands for 30 to 45 minutes

Wednesday
- Naked Get-Ups for five minutes
- Mobility Sequence
- Practice a few Hip Hinge Drills and a few Goblet Squat prying movements.
- Do three to five sets of presses and squats (Reps as appropriate; stop when you have two to five reps still "in the pocket.")
- Bearpees (If you want some extra conditioning)
- Walk

Thursday
- GetBackUps
- Mobility Sequence for 30-60 minutes

Friday
(This day can be swapped with Saturday if one prefers to train on the weekends.)
- Naked Turkish Get-Ups for five minutes
- Mobility Sequence
- Practice a few Hip Hinge Drills and a few Goblet Squat prying movements.
- Humane Burpee or Armor Building Challenge
- Turkish Get-Ups, one to five per side.
- Cook Drill
- Walk

Saturday
- Long Walk, Hike, Walk, or Bike

Sunday
- It's an off day or anything you wish to do.

Week Two

Monday
- Naked Get-Ups for five minutes
- Mobility Sequence
- Practice a few Hip Hinge Drills and a few Goblet Squat prying movements.
- Do three to five sets of presses and squats (Reps as appropriate; stop when you have two to five reps still "in the pocket.")
- Bearpees (If you wish more conditioning)
- Walk

Tuesday
- GetBackUps
- Mobility Sequence
- Walk, Ruck, or HeavyHands for 30 to 45 minutes

Wednesday
- Naked Get-Ups for five minutes
- Mobility Sequence
- Practice a few Hip Hinge Drills and a few Goblet Squat prying movements.
- Humane Burpee or Armor Building Challenge
- Turkish Get-Ups, one to five per side.
- Cook Drill
- Walk

Thursday
- GetBackUps
- Mobility Sequence for 30-60 minutes

Friday
(This day can be swapped with Saturday if one prefers to train on the weekends.)
- Naked Get-Ups for five minutes
- Mobility Sequence
- Practice a few Hip Hinge Drills and a few Goblet Squat prying movements.
- Do three to five sets of presses and squats (Reps as appropriate; stop when you have two to five reps still "in the pocket.")
- Hornees (if you wish more conditioning)
- Walk

Saturday
- Long Walk, Hike, Walk, or Bike

Sunday
- It's an off day or anything you wish to do.

The Advanced Kettlebell Hypertrophy Program

Finally, let me share an advanced program we use for a kettlebell-focused hypertrophy and strength phase. Again, some of the exercises are just names we use; I share most of them on my YouTube channel. Don't worry about the specifics too much; get a sense of the whole program.

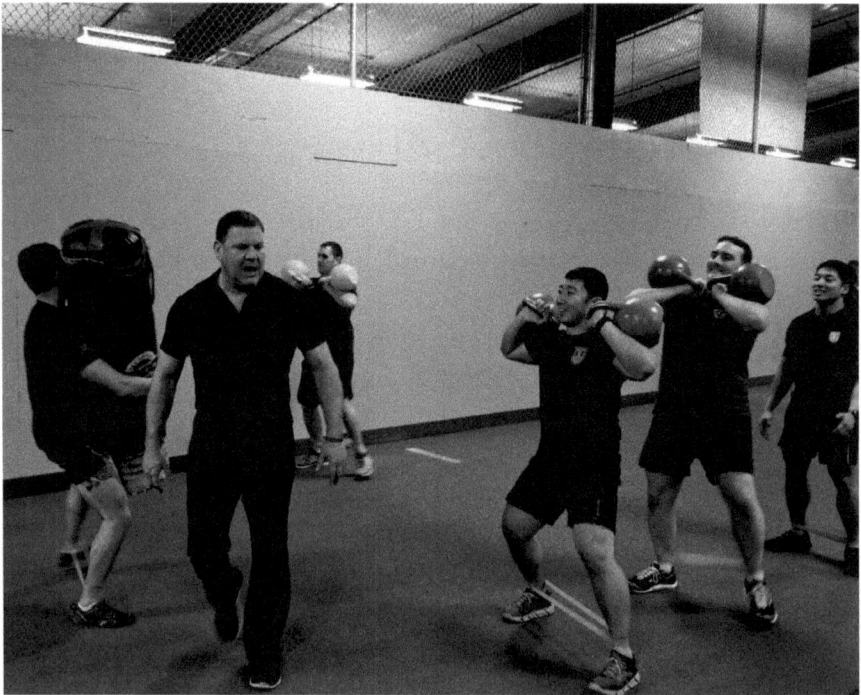

Dan "helping" the Green Berets learn this workout.

Monday

Naked Get-Ups
15 Swings/5 Goblet Squat/March in Place
Stoney Stretch (RKD)
15 Swings/4 Goblet Squat/March in Place
Windmill Stick "Look Right
15 Swings/3 Goblet Squat/March in Place
Naked Get-Ups
15 Swings/2 Goblet Squat/March in Place
Stoney Stretch (LKD)
15 Swings/I Goblet Squat/March in Place
Windmill Stick "Look Left"
Subtotal:
Hinge: 75
Squat: 15

Two Times
25 Hip Thrusts
5 Double Kettlebell Front Squats
15 Swings
Mini-Band Walk
Farmer Walk

Pull-Ups: 3-2-2-2-1
One-Arm Press: 1-1-1-1-1

Two Rounds of
TRX T x 25
Ab Wheel x 5

25 Hip Thrust
10 Swings plus 5/4/3/2/1/ Goblet Squats

Push: 5
Pull: 60
Hinge: 230
Squat: 40
Two Loaded Carry Variations
Four Sixth Movements

Tuesday

Naked Get-Ups
Hip Thrusts x 10/15 Swings/5 Goblet Squat/March in Place
Stoney Stretch (RKD)
Hip Thrusts x 10/15 Swings/4 Goblet Squat/March in Place
Windmill Stick "Look Right
Hip Thrusts x 10/15 Swings/3 Goblet Squat/March in Place
Naked Get-Ups
Hip Thrusts x 10/15 Swings/2 Goblet Squat/March in Place
Stoney Stretch (LKD)
Hip Thrusts x 10/15 Swings/I Goblet Squat/March in Place
Windmill Stick "Look Left"
Subtotal:
Hinge: 125
Squat: 15

Three Circuits:

8 x T-Y-I Row
5 Ab Wheel Roll Out
Hip Rip R/L

Pull-Ups: 3-3-2-2-1
One-Arm Press: 2-1-1-1-1

Three Circuits
TRX Biceps Curl x 15
TRX Triceps Extension x 15

Bear Crawl-Bear Hug with Sandbag (or other load) x 2

Push: 6 (45 Extensions)
Pull: 83
Hinge: 125
Squat: 15
Loaded Carry: Two Variations
Four Sixth Movements

Thursday

Naked Get-Ups
Hip Thrusts x 10/15 Swings/5 Goblet Squat/March in Place
Stoney Stretch (RKD)
Hip Thrusts x 10/15 Swings/4 Goblet Squat/March in Place
Windmill Stick "Look Right
Hip Thrusts x 10/15 Swings/3 Goblet Squat/March in Place
Naked Get-Ups
Hip Thrusts x 10/15 Swings/2 Goblet Squat/March in Place
Stoney Stretch (LKD)
Hip Thrusts x 10/15 Swings/I Goblet Squat/March in Place
Windmill Stick "Look Left"
Subtotal:
Hinge: 125
Squat: 15

Pull-Ups: 3-3-3-2-1
One-Arm Press: 2-2-1-1-1

Double KB Press
2-3-5-10 (Finish all twenty reps before moving on to the Hip Thrusts)
Between sets, do Rocks, Hip Flexor Stretch, and be a general nuisance

Hip Thrust x 25
Goblet Squat x 10
Suitcase Carry
Three Total Rounds. Round One: Light Double Presses. Round Two: Heavy Double Presses. Round Three: Medium Double Press

Push: 67
Pull: 12
Hinge: 200
Squat: 45
Loaded Carry: One Variation
Four Sixth Movements

Friday

Naked Get-Ups
15 Swings/5 Goblet Squat/March in Place
Stoney Stretch (RKD)
15 Swings/4 Goblet Squat/March in Place
Windmill Stick "Look Right
15 Swings/3 Goblet Squat/March in Place
Naked Get-Ups
15 Swings/2 Goblet Squat/March in Place
Stoney Stretch (LKD)
15 Swings/I Goblet Squat/March in Place
Windmill Stick "Look Left"
Subtotal:
Hinge: 75
Squat: 15

Pull-Ups: 1-1-1
One-Arm Press: 1-1-1

Mini-Band Walk with Black
Double KB Front Squat x 3
Waiter Walk

Double KB Front Squat x 3
Farmer Walk
Double KB Front Squat x 3
Light Bag Carry
Double KB Front Squat x 3
Medium Bag Carry
Double KB Front Squat x 3
Heavy Bag Carry
Double KB Front Squat x 3

Two Rounds
TRX Triceps Extension x 15
TRX Biceps Curls x 15
KB French Press x 15
Barbell Curls x 15

Push: 3 (plus 30 Extensions)
Pull: 3
Hinge: 75
Squat: 33
Loaded Carry: Six Variations
Two Sixth Movements

Weekly Numbers:

Push: 81 (Plus all the Extensions)
Pull: 158
Hinge: 605
Squat: 133
Loaded Carries: 11 Variations
Sixth Movements: 14 Variations

The Twelve Days of Kettlebells: A Summary

The Twelve Levels of Training to Explore
- "Earth:" On your back, Prone, Six Point, Bear, Half-kneeling
- "Human:" Squat, Hinge, Gait, Carry
- "Sky:" Air, Hang, Brachiate

The Eleven Truths of Longevity
- Go to bed two hours after sundown (as appropriate)
- Wake up and move
- Never hit the snooze button
- Wear your seatbelt (and helmet)
- Don't smoke
- Learn to fall and recover
- Floss (!!!)
- 100 minutes of exercise a week (This is the minimum)
- Stay "knitted:" Be part of a community (Ideally, communities!)
- Keep your weight under 300 pounds (138 kilograms)
- Eat protein and veggies. Drink water.

The Ten Commandments of "Keeping the Goal the Goal" as a Coach
- Train appropriate to your goal(s).
- Train "little and often over the long haul."
- The longer it takes to get in shape or condition, the "longer" the shape or condition remains.
- Warm-up and cool-down really have a role.
- Be sure to train for volume before you train for intensity.
- You must cycle the workouts somehow.
- Train in a community, of some kind.
- Train your mind.

- Keep your training program in perspective.
- Yes, the Fundamentals (the basics) will rule everything else: fundamental movements, the basics of flexibility and mobility, basic techniques, and basic nutrition.

The Nine Key Muscle Groups... *for most of us*
Strengthen these:
- Glutes
- Rhomboids
- Deltoids
- Triceps
- Abs

> **Yes, the Fundamentals (the basics) will rule everything else.**

Stretch these:
- Pectorals
- Biceps
- Hamstrings
- Hip Flexors

(Taken from the work of Vlad Janda, I find this a simple way to organize most programming for Americans)

The Eight Not-So-Secret Secrets of Nutrition (Diet)
- Eat like an adult
- Focus on protein and vegetables
- Drink water
- Avoid drinking calories
- Train in a fasted state sometimes
- Stay hungry after some workouts
- Food (including fermented foods and fruit) are probably the best supplements
- Nutrition has never been complicated, but "simple" makes it harder to make money

The Seven Tools to Teach "Stay Tall"
- Push-Up Position Plank
- Vertical Plank
- Goblet Squat
- Farmer Walk
- Suitcase Carry
- Deadlift
- March in Place with High Knees

The Basic Kettlebell Six
- Snatch
- Clean
- Press
- Goblet Squat
- Swing
- Get-Up

The Five Fundamental Human Movements (Weightroom Edition)
- Push
- Pull
- Hinge
- Squat
- Loaded Carries

The Four Points of the LIFE Compass
- Work
- Rest
- Play
- Pray

Take a moment daily to ensure that your work, rest, play, and pray (including quality alone time, enjoying nature and art, and avoiding social media and "noise" for a bit) remain in a healthy, reasonable balance.

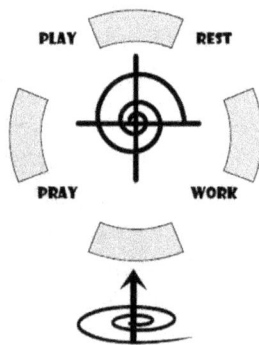

The Hardstyle Kettlebell Three
- Goblet Squat
- Swing
- Get-Up

The Daily "Do This!" Mobility Two
- 30 seconds of hanging from a bar
- 30 seconds of sitting in the bottom of the Goblet Squat

The Body is One Piece
One can't separate their emotional issues from physical issues from work and life and family issues from spiritual issues from financial issues from...we are ONE PIECE!

Never Let Go!

Learn More

COACH
DAN JOHN

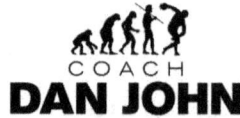

Dan John has been lifting since 1965 and has won national championships in the discus throw, Olympic lifting, Highland Games, and the Weight Pentathlon. He was recently awarded a Lifetime Achievement Award from Great Britain for his contributions to the field of strength and conditioning. A Fulbright Scholar, he has vast experience in scholarship, academics, and athletics. Dan has advanced degrees in history and religious education and has studied at the University of Haifa, the American University of Cairo, and Cornell. He is a former Senior Lecturer at Saint Mary's University in Twickenham, England.

His books include bestsellers such as Easy Strength Omnibook, Never Let Go, Mass Made Simple, and Intervention (among almost two dozen other published works) and countless articles. He is the grandfather to five and continues to write, coach, train, and lecture to practically every fitness and performance level.

His website is https://danjohnuniversity.com/

Enjoy his YouTube channel at
https://www.youtube.com/@DanJohnStrengthCoach

Find him on Instagram at https://www.instagram.com/coachdanjohn/